THE ANATOMY OF YOGA

How To Improve Your Balance, Strength And Mobility In Few Days With Yoga

DR. ARTHUR STEVES

TABLE OF CONTENTS

CHAPTER 5 40

CHAPTER 6 50

CHAPTER 7 58

CHAPTER 11 92

CHAPTER 12 100

INTRODUCTION TO YOGA ANATOMY

Yoga is a practice that integrates the mind, body, and spirit through physical postures (asanas), breath control (pranayama), and meditation. While yoga is often celebrated for its mental and spiritual benefits, the physical practice plays a crucial role in enhancing overall well-being. Understanding the anatomy of yoga is essential for anyone looking to deepen their practice, whether they are a beginner, a seasoned practitioner, or a yoga teacher.

Yoga anatomy focuses on the interaction between the body's musculoskeletal system and the movements performed during yoga practice. By understanding how muscles, bones, joints, and connective tissues work together, practitioners can improve their posture, flexibility, strength, and balance. Knowledge of anatomy helps in:

Preventing Injuries: Recognizing the limitations of your body and understanding the mechanics of each pose can prevent overextension, strain, and injury.

Enhancing Performance: Knowing which muscles to engage and how to align the body properly in each pose can improve the effectiveness of the practice, leading to greater physical benefits.

Promoting Healing: Yoga can be therapeutic, and understanding anatomy allows for modifications and adaptations to suit individual needs, especially during recovery from injuries or managing chronic conditions.

Yoga is more than just a series of physical exercises; it is a holistic practice that impacts the entire body. To fully appreciate how yoga affects the body, it's important to have a basic understanding of the following systems:

Musculoskeletal System: This system includes bones, muscles, tendons, ligaments, and fascia. Yoga poses (asanas) directly impact this system by stretching and strengthening muscles, improving joint mobility, and enhancing overall structural alignment.

Nervous System: Yoga has a profound effect on the nervous system, helping to calm the mind, reduce stress, and improve mental clarity. The practice of pranayama (breathing techniques) and meditation also positively affects the nervous system by regulating the body's response to stress.

Respiratory System: Breath is a central component of yoga practice. Understanding the anatomy of the respiratory system helps in mastering pranayama techniques, which are essential for enhancing lung capacity, improving oxygen intake, and balancing the body's energy.

Circulatory System: Yoga promotes better circulation by encouraging movement, deep breathing, and relaxation. Certain poses can help increase blood flow to specific areas of the body, aiding in the delivery of oxygen and nutrients to tissues and the removal of waste products.

Digestive System: Many yoga poses are designed to stimulate and support the digestive system. Twists, in particular, are known for their ability to massage the internal organs, aiding in digestion and detoxification.

Endocrine System: Yoga helps regulate the endocrine system, which controls hormones that affect mood, energy levels, metabolism, and other bodily functions. Specific poses can stimulate different glands, helping to balance hormone production.

Understanding anatomy allows yoga practitioners to approach their practice with greater mindfulness and intention. Rather than simply going through the motions of each pose, practitioners can focus on:

Alignment: Proper alignment is key to a safe and effective yoga practice. By aligning the body correctly, practitioners can reduce strain on the joints and muscles, ensuring that the benefits of each pose are maximized.

Breath Awareness: The breath is a powerful tool in yoga. By coordinating breath with movement, practitioners can improve their focus, deepen their poses, and create a sense of harmony between mind and body.

Body Awareness: Developing a keen awareness of the body's capabilities and limitations is crucial in yoga. Understanding anatomy helps practitioners listen to their bodies, make necessary adjustments, and avoid pushing beyond their limits.

Informed Adjustments: For yoga teachers, knowledge of anatomy is essential for providing safe and effective adjustments to students. By understanding how different bodies move, teachers can offer personalized guidance that respects each student's unique anatomy.

In conclusion, yoga anatomy is not just for teachers or advanced practitioners—it is for anyone who wants to practice yoga safely and effectively. Whether you are looking to deepen your practice, prevent injuries, or simply gain a better understanding of your body, exploring the anatomy of yoga is a vital step on your journey.

CHAPTER 1

The Muscular System in Yoga

The muscular system is fundamental to the practice of yoga, as it plays a crucial role in movement, stability, and overall physical function. Understanding how muscles work during yoga poses allows practitioners to engage them more effectively, enhance their practice, and avoid injury.

Understanding Muscle Function in Yoga

Muscles are responsible for producing movement by contracting and generating force, which is then transferred to the bones through tendons. In yoga, different muscle groups work together to create, control, and stabilize movements. The three primary functions of muscles in yoga are:

Contraction: Muscles contract to create movement. There are three types of muscle contractions:

Isotonic Contraction: The muscle changes length during the contraction, leading to movement. This includes concentric (shortening) and eccentric (lengthening) contractions.

Isometric Contraction: The muscle length remains constant while contracting, maintaining a position without movement. This is common in poses like Plank (Phalakasana) where muscles work to stabilize the body.

Relaxation: After contracting, muscles relax, allowing for lengthening or resting. Proper relaxation is essential for flexibility and recovery.

Stabilization: Muscles also work to stabilize the body, particularly in balancing poses. Core muscles, for example, stabilize the spine and pelvis in many yoga postures.

Major Muscle Groups in Common Yoga Poses
In yoga, various muscle groups are activated depending on the pose. Here are some key muscle groups and their roles in common yoga asanas:

Core Muscles
Rectus Abdominis: Known as the "six-pack," this muscle flexes the spine and stabilizes the pelvis. It is engaged in poses like Boat Pose (Navasana) and Plank (Phalakasana).

Transverse Abdominis: The deepest abdominal muscle, it acts like a corset, stabilizing the spine and pelvis. It's crucial for maintaining stability in most yoga poses.

Obliques: These muscles run along the sides of the abdomen, aiding in twisting poses like Revolved Triangle Pose (Parivrtta Trikonasana).

Back Muscles

Erector Spinae: These muscles run along the spine, helping with spinal extension and maintaining posture. They are engaged in backbends like Cobra Pose (Bhujangasana) and Locust Pose (Salabhasana).

Latissimus Dorsi: This broad back muscle assists in arm movements and is engaged in poses like Downward Dog (Adho Mukha Svanasana) and Warrior II (Virabhadrasana II).

Leg Muscles

Quadriceps: Located at the front of the thigh, these muscles extend the knee and are engaged in poses like Warrior I (Virabhadrasana I) and Chair Pose (Utkatasana).

Hamstrings: These muscles run along the back of the thigh and are responsible for knee flexion and hip extension. They are stretched in Forward Fold (Uttanasana) and engaged in Bridge Pose (Setu Bandhasana).

Gluteus Maximus: This powerful muscle in the buttocks is engaged in hip extension, as in poses like Warrior III (Virabhadrasana III) and Bridge Pose (Setu Bandhasana).

Adductors: Inner thigh muscles that bring the legs together, essential for maintaining stability in poses like Tree Pose (Vrksasana).

Arm and Shoulder Muscles

Deltoids: These muscles cover the shoulder and are responsible for lifting and rotating the arm. They are engaged in poses like Downward Dog (Adho Mukha Svanasana) and Crow Pose (Bakasana).

Biceps and Triceps: The biceps flex the elbow, while the triceps extend it. Both are engaged in arm-balancing poses like Chaturanga Dandasana and Side Plank (Vasisthasana).

Rotator Cuff Muscles: A group of muscles that stabilize the shoulder joint, crucial in poses requiring arm strength and stability, such as Dolphin Pose (Ardha Pincha Mayurasana).

Muscle Engagement and Relaxation Techniques

Proper muscle engagement and relaxation are vital for safe and effective yoga practice. Here are some techniques to optimize muscle use in yoga:

Engage the Core: Activating the core muscles stabilizes the spine and pelvis, providing a strong foundation for most poses. To engage the core, draw the navel toward the spine and maintain this activation throughout the practice.

Use Isometric Contractions: In poses where stability is key, such as Warrior Poses or Plank, engage muscles isometrically. This involves contracting muscles without changing their length, maintaining the pose with strength and control.

Balance Strength and Flexibility: Yoga requires both muscle strength and flexibility. In poses that involve stretching, like Forward Folds or Backbends, focus on engaging the opposing muscle groups to protect joints and prevent overstretching.

Practice Relaxation: Equally important as engagement is the ability to relax muscles when needed. In restorative poses or Savasana (Corpse Pose), allow muscles to fully release and relax, promoting recovery and mental calm.

Common Misconceptions about Muscles in Yoga
More Stretching Equals More Flexibility: While stretching muscles is important, flexibility also requires muscle strength and proper alignment. Overstretching without engaging the opposing muscles can lead to injury.

Yoga is Only for Flexibility: Yoga builds both strength and flexibility. Many poses, especially arm balances and standing poses, require significant muscle strength.

Muscle Engagement Means Tension: Engaging muscles doesn't mean creating unnecessary tension. The goal is to engage muscles mindfully and with control, maintaining balance and ease in each pose.

Understanding the muscular system in yoga empowers practitioners to enhance their practice, achieve better alignment, and develop both strength and flexibility. By consciously engaging and relaxing muscles, practitioners can move through poses with greater awareness and effectiveness.

CHAPTER 2
The Skeletal System and Joint Anatomy

The skeletal system provides the structural framework for the body, supporting movement, protecting vital organs, and storing essential minerals. In yoga, understanding the skeletal system and joint anatomy is crucial for proper alignment, safe practice, and effective movement. This knowledge allows practitioners to move with greater awareness and helps prevent injuries.

The Role of Bones in Supporting Yoga Postures

Bones are the rigid structures that make up the skeleton, providing the body with shape and support. They serve as attachment points for muscles, enabling movement through joints. In yoga, bones:

Support Weight: In standing and balancing poses, bones bear the body's weight, helping maintain stability.

Provide Structure: Bones determine the body's shape and form, influencing how a practitioner moves through and holds different yoga poses.

Act as Levers: Bones act as levers that muscles pull on to create movement, allowing the body to perform various yoga asanas.

Understanding Joint Mechanics

Joints are where two or more bones meet, allowing for movement and flexibility. Different types of joints permit varying degrees of motion, and understanding their mechanics helps in practicing yoga safely and effectively. The major types of joints relevant to yoga practice include:

Hinge Joints

Examples: Knees, Elbows
Movement: Hinge joints allow movement in one plane, like a door hinge, permitting flexion (bending) and extension (straightening).
Yoga Poses: In poses like Downward Dog (Adho Mukha Svanasana) and Plank (Phalakasana), hinge joints must be properly aligned to avoid hyperextension or strain.

Ball-and-Socket Joints

Examples: Shoulders, Hips
Movement: These joints allow for movement in multiple directions, including flexion, extension, abduction, adduction, and rotation.
Yoga Poses: In poses like Warrior II (Virabhadrasana II) and Tree Pose (Vrksasana), proper alignment of the hips and shoulders is crucial to protect these versatile joints from injury.

Pivot Joints

Examples: Neck (Atlantoaxial Joint)

Movement: Pivot joints allow for rotation around a single axis.

Yoga Poses: In poses involving neck rotation, like Half Lord of the Fishes Pose (Ardha Matsyendrasana), awareness of the pivot joint in the neck helps in maintaining safe and controlled movement.

Ellipsoid Joints

Examples: Wrists

Movement: Ellipsoid joints permit movement in two planes, allowing for flexion, extension, abduction, and adduction.

Yoga Poses: In arm balances like Crow Pose (Bakasana), wrist alignment is critical to prevent strain or injury.

Saddle Joints

Examples: Thumb

Movement: Saddle joints allow for movement in multiple directions, similar to a ball-and-socket joint but with less range.

Yoga Poses: Thumb engagement and positioning in poses that require hand balance, like Downward Dog, is essential for stability.

Plane (Gliding) Joints

Examples: Carpals of the Wrist, Tarsals of the Feet

Movement: These joints allow for limited movement in various directions, as the bones glide past each other.
Yoga Poses: Awareness of plane joints helps in poses that require precise hand and foot placement, like in Plank or Standing Forward Bend (Uttanasana).
Spine: The Central Support

The spine, or vertebral column, is a crucial element in yoga practice, providing both support and flexibility. It is composed of 33 vertebrae divided into five regions:

Cervical Spine (Neck)
Function: Supports the head and allows for a wide range of motion.
Yoga Consideration: In poses like Shoulder Stand (Sarvangasana) or Headstand (Sirsasana), it's important to maintain alignment to protect the cervical spine from compression.
Thoracic Spine (Upper Back)

Function: Anchors the ribcage and supports the upper body.
Yoga Consideration: This part of the spine has limited flexibility, so in backbends like Camel Pose (Ustrasana), the movement should come more from the lumbar spine to avoid straining the thoracic area.

Lumbar Spine (Lower Back)

Function: Bears much of the body's weight and allows for flexion and extension.

Yoga Consideration: In forward bends like Seated Forward Bend (Paschimottanasana), it's crucial to hinge from the hips rather than rounding the lumbar spine to prevent injury.

Sacral Spine (Pelvic Area)

Function: Transmits weight from the upper body to the pelvis and legs.

Yoga Consideration: Awareness of the sacrum's position helps in poses like Warrior I (Virabhadrasana I), ensuring proper pelvic alignment.

Coccyx (Tailbone)

Function: Provides attachment for ligaments and muscles of the pelvic floor.

Yoga Consideration: The coccyx should be gently tucked in poses like Mountain Pose (Tadasana) to support proper spinal alignment.

Shoulders and Hips: Ball-and-Socket Joints

The shoulders and hips are the body's most mobile joints, allowing for a wide range of movement. However, this mobility also makes them vulnerable to injury if not properly aligned in yoga poses.

Shoulders: In poses like Downward Dog (Adho Mukha Svanasana) or Upward Dog (Urdhva Mukha Svanasana), it's essential to stabilize the shoulder blades and avoid excessive elevation or internal rotation, which can strain the rotator cuff muscles.

Hips: In poses like Warrior II (Virabhadrasana II) or Pigeon Pose (Eka Pada Rajakapotasana), proper hip alignment is key to avoiding stress on the hip joint and associated muscles, like the hip flexors and glutes.

Knees and Elbows: Hinge Joints

Knees and elbows are hinge joints that only allow for flexion and extension. Due to their limited range of motion, they require careful attention during yoga practice.

Knees: In poses like Warrior I (Virabhadrasana I) or Chair Pose (Utkatasana), ensure that the knee aligns over the ankle, and avoid letting it extend past the toes to prevent strain on the ligaments and tendons.

Elbows: In Chaturanga Dandasana or Plank Pose, it's important to keep the elbows close to the body and slightly bent to avoid hyperextension and maintain joint stability.

Safe Joint Alignment and Injury Prevention

Proper joint alignment is vital for a safe and sustainable yoga practice. Misalignment can lead to joint wear and tear, discomfort, and injuries over time. Here are some tips for maintaining safe joint alignment:

Listen to Your Body: Respect your body's limits and avoid forcing movements that cause pain or discomfort. Use props or modify poses as needed to support your joints.

Engage Muscles to Support Joints: Use the surrounding muscles to stabilize joints in all poses. For example, engage the quadriceps to protect the knees in standing poses.

Maintain Neutral Alignment: In poses like Tadasana (Mountain Pose), ensure that the joints are stacked, with the hips over the knees and the knees over the ankles. This alignment helps distribute weight evenly and reduces joint stress.

Avoid Hyperextension: Be mindful of locking the joints, particularly in the knees and elbows. Slightly bend these joints to engage the surrounding muscles and protect the ligaments.

Warm Up Properly: Before attempting deeper stretches or challenging poses, take time to warm up the body, focusing on gentle movements that increase blood flow to the joints.

Understanding the skeletal system and joint anatomy is foundational for practicing yoga with awareness and precision. By aligning the bones and supporting the joints with proper muscle engagement, practitioners can enhance their practice, prevent injuries, and achieve a deeper connection with their bodies.

CHAPTER 3

Connective Tissues in Yoga

Connective tissues play a crucial role in the practice of yoga, as they provide structure, support, and stability to the body. These tissues include ligaments, tendons, and fascia, all of which are integral to the movement and alignment of the body in yoga postures. Understanding the anatomy and function of connective tissues allows practitioners to approach their practice with greater awareness, improving flexibility, strength, and overall well-being.

Ligaments and Their Role in Joint Stability

Ligaments are tough, fibrous tissues that connect bones to other bones at joints, providing stability and guiding joint movement. In yoga, ligaments are essential for:

Stabilizing Joints: Ligaments prevent excessive movement that could lead to joint dislocation or injury. For example, the knee ligaments help stabilize the knee during poses like Warrior II (Virabhadrasana II).

Limiting Range of Motion: While ligaments allow for normal joint movement, they also limit the range to prevent hyperextension or hyperflexion. In yoga, it's important not to push the joints beyond their natural range, as overstretching ligaments can lead to instability and injury.

Yoga Considerations for Ligament Health:
Avoid Overstretching: Ligaments are not as elastic as muscles and do not easily return to their original length if overstretched. Practitioners should be cautious in deep stretches and avoid pushing beyond their flexibility limits.

Focus on Joint Alignment: Proper alignment in poses helps distribute forces evenly across the ligaments, reducing the risk of strain. For example, in Triangle Pose (Trikonasana), aligning the knee over the ankle protects the ligaments in the knee joint.

Tendons and Muscle-Bone Connection
Tendons are strong, fibrous cords that connect muscles to bones, transmitting the force generated by muscle contraction to the skeleton to create movement. In yoga, tendons are key to:

Facilitating Movement: Tendons transmit the force from muscle contractions to bones, enabling movement in yoga poses. For example, the Achilles tendon connects the calf muscles to the heel bone, playing a crucial role in poses like Downward Dog (Adho Mukha Svanasana).
Absorbing Impact: Tendons absorb some of the impact from dynamic movements, helping to protect muscles and joints from injury.

Yoga Considerations for Tendon Health:
Gradual Progression: Tendons adapt to stress more slowly than muscles, so it's important to progress gradually in yoga practice to avoid tendon strain. Incorporating warm-up exercises and gradually increasing the intensity of stretches can help protect tendons.

Balance Strength and Flexibility: Strengthening the muscles surrounding a tendon can help protect it from injury. For instance, strengthening the hamstrings can support the tendons in the back of the knee during poses like Warrior III (Virabhadrasana III).

The Fascial System: Structure and Function
Fascia is a web-like network of connective tissue that surrounds and supports muscles, bones, and organs throughout the body. It plays a vital role in maintaining structural integrity, facilitating movement, and transmitting force. In yoga, fascia is involved in:

Supporting Movement: Fascia connects different parts of the body, allowing for coordinated movement. For example, the fascia connects the muscles along the back of the body, playing a key role in forward bends and backbends.

Transmitting Force: Fascia helps distribute the force of movement throughout the body, reducing the risk of injury. In yoga, this means that stretching one part of the body can have effects elsewhere, emphasizing the importance of holistic movement.

Providing Structural Integrity: Fascia helps maintain the body's shape and structure. It also influences posture and movement patterns, making it a key focus in yoga practice.

Yoga Considerations for Fascial Health:

Practice Mindful Movement: Fascia responds well to slow, mindful movement, which helps it remain pliable and healthy. Gentle stretching and flowing movements, as found in Vinyasa yoga, can help keep the fascia flexible.

Hydration and Recovery: Fascia needs to be hydrated to function properly. Adequate hydration and rest between yoga sessions help maintain fascial health and prevent stiffness.

Addressing Fascial Restrictions: Areas of tight fascia can create tension and restrict movement. Techniques such as myofascial release (using foam rollers or massage balls) can help release these restrictions and improve flexibility.

Techniques to Improve Fascia Health

Maintaining healthy fascia is essential for flexibility, mobility, and overall physical well-being. In yoga, there are several techniques that can help improve the health of the fascial system:

Slow, Sustained Stretches

Yin Yoga: This style of yoga involves holding poses for extended periods, which helps to gently stretch and hydrate the fascia. Poses like Butterfly (Baddha Konasana) and Sphinx (Salamba Bhujangasana) are examples of Yin poses that target fascia.

Dynamic Movements

Flow Yoga: Dynamic, flowing movements, such as in Vinyasa yoga, help to keep the fascia supple and prevent it from becoming too rigid. These movements also promote the circulation of synovial fluid, which lubricates the joints and fascia.

Myofascial Release

Self-Massage Tools: Using tools like foam rollers or massage balls can help release tension in the fascia. Rolling out areas like the IT band (along the outer thigh) or the soles of the feet can alleviate tightness and improve mobility.

Hydration

Stay Hydrated: Drinking plenty of water is essential for keeping the fascia hydrated and healthy. Dehydrated fascia becomes stiff and less pliable, which can limit movement and increase the risk of injury.

Mind-Body Connection

Body Awareness Practices: Incorporating mindfulness and body awareness into your yoga practice helps you tune into areas of tightness or restriction in the fascia. Gentle movements and stretches can then be used to release these areas.

Understanding and caring for the connective tissues is crucial for a balanced and sustainable yoga practice. By paying attention to ligaments, tendons, and fascia, practitioners can enhance their flexibility, improve joint stability, and reduce the risk of injury. Integrating knowledge of connective tissues into your yoga practice fosters a deeper connection with your body and promotes long-term physical health.

CHAPTER 4

The Nervous System and Yoga

The nervous system plays a vital role in yoga, as it governs the body's response to stress, movement, and relaxation. By understanding how the nervous system functions and interacts with the body during yoga practice, practitioners can enhance their ability to manage stress, improve mental clarity, and deepen their mind-body connection.

Overview of the Nervous System

The nervous system is a complex network that controls and coordinates all bodily functions. It is divided into two main parts:

Central Nervous System (CNS)

Components: The CNS consists of the brain and spinal cord.

Function: It processes and interprets sensory information and sends out instructions to the body. The CNS is the command center for all mental and physical activities.

Peripheral Nervous System (PNS)

Components: The PNS includes all the nerves that branch out from the spinal cord and brain, extending to the rest of the body.

Function: The PNS carries messages between the CNS and the body. It is further divided into the somatic nervous system (voluntary control) and the autonomic nervous system (involuntary control).

The Autonomic Nervous System (ANS) is particularly important in yoga, as it regulates involuntary body functions such as heart rate, digestion, and respiration. The ANS has two main branches:

Sympathetic Nervous System (SNS): Known as the "fight-or-flight" system, the SNS prepares the body for stressful situations by increasing heart rate, dilating airways, and releasing stress hormones.

Parasympathetic Nervous System (PNS): Known as the "rest-and-digest" system, the PNS promotes relaxation, digestion, and recovery by slowing the heart rate, constricting airways, and encouraging calmness.

Yoga's Impact on the Nervous System

Yoga can have profound effects on the nervous system, particularly in balancing the SNS and PNS. Through various practices such as breath control (pranayama), meditation, and physical postures (asanas), yoga helps to modulate the nervous system, leading to improved physical and mental health.

Pranayama (Breath Control)

Influence on the Nervous System: Pranayama techniques directly affect the autonomic nervous system by regulating the breath. Deep, slow breathing stimulates the PNS, promoting relaxation and reducing stress. Practices like Ujjayi breathing and Nadi Shodhana (alternate nostril breathing) can help calm the mind and balance the nervous system. Example: Slow, deep diaphragmatic breathing, commonly used in yoga, activates the vagus nerve, which is a key component of the PNS. This leads to a reduction in heart rate and blood pressure, helping the body shift into a state of relaxation.

Asanas (Physical Postures)

Influence on the Nervous System: Physical postures in yoga help to release tension in the body, improve circulation, and balance the nervous system. Certain poses stimulate the SNS, energizing the body, while others activate the PNS, promoting relaxation.
Example: Inversions like Shoulder Stand (Sarvangasana) can stimulate the PNS by increasing blood flow to the brain, which can have a calming effect. Conversely, poses like Warrior II (Virabhadrasana II) can stimulate the SNS, providing a sense of strength and alertness.

Meditation and Mindfulness

Influence on the Nervous System: Meditation practices in yoga promote mindfulness, reduce stress, and enhance the connection between the mind and body. Regular meditation helps to downregulate the SNS and enhance the activity of the PNS, leading to improved emotional regulation and mental clarity.

Example: Mindfulness meditation, where one focuses on the present moment without judgment, has been shown to reduce the activity of the amygdala (the brain's stress response center) and increase activity in the prefrontal cortex (associated with calmness and focus).

Yoga Nidra (Yogic Sleep)

Influence on the Nervous System: Yoga Nidra is a form of guided meditation that leads to deep relaxation and is often referred to as "yogic sleep." It promotes a state between wakefulness and sleep, activating the PNS and allowing the body and mind to rest deeply.

Example: During Yoga Nidra, the body enters a state of deep relaxation, which helps reduce the production of stress hormones like cortisol. This practice can be particularly beneficial for those experiencing chronic stress or anxiety.

The Stress Response and Yoga

The stress response, primarily governed by the SNS, is the body's natural reaction to perceived threats. While this response is essential for survival, chronic activation of the SNS can lead to health issues such as anxiety, insomnia, high blood pressure, and weakened immune function. Yoga helps to mitigate the effects of chronic stress by:

Reducing Cortisol Levels: Regular yoga practice has been shown to lower cortisol levels, the body's primary stress hormone. Lower cortisol levels are associated with reduced stress, improved mood, and better immune function.

Enhancing Resilience: By regularly practicing yoga, individuals can improve their ability to manage stress, leading to a more balanced and resilient nervous system. This helps in responding to stressful situations with greater calmness and control.

Neuroplasticity and Yoga
Neuroplasticity refers to the brain's ability to reorganize itself by forming new neural connections throughout life. Yoga, particularly through meditation and mindful movement, can enhance neuroplasticity by:

Improving Cognitive Function: Meditation and mindfulness practices in yoga have been shown to increase gray matter in areas of the brain associated with memory, learning, and emotional regulation.
Promoting Emotional Balance: By regularly engaging in yoga, practitioners can improve their emotional regulation and reduce the impact of negative emotions. This is partly due to the effects of yoga on neuroplasticity, which allows for the rewiring of negative thought patterns into more positive ones.

Balancing the Nervous System Through Yoga

To maintain a balanced nervous system, it's essential to incorporate a variety of yoga practices that both stimulate and relax the body and mind. Here are some approaches to achieve this balance:

Alternate Stimulation and Relaxation:

Energizing Practices: Incorporate dynamic practices like Sun Salutations (Surya Namaskar) or Vinyasa flows to stimulate the SNS and increase energy levels.

Relaxing Practices: Follow up with restorative poses, gentle stretching, or meditation to activate the PNS and promote relaxation.

Focus on Breath Awareness:

Breath Control: Use pranayama techniques to consciously regulate the breath, helping to shift the balance between the SNS and PNS. For example, lengthening the exhalation relative to the inhalation can enhance PNS activity and promote relaxation.

Practice Regular Meditation:

Mindfulness Meditation: Engage in daily meditation practices to cultivate awareness, reduce stress, and improve mental clarity. Even a few minutes of meditation each day can have significant benefits for the nervous system.

Incorporate Restorative Yoga:

Restorative Poses: Include restorative poses such as Child's Pose (Balasana), Legs Up the Wall (Viparita Karani), and Savasana (Corpse Pose) to allow the nervous system to rest and recover.

Engage in Yoga Nidra:
Deep Relaxation: Practice Yoga Nidra regularly to promote deep relaxation and activate the PNS, allowing the body and mind to heal and rejuvenate.

By understanding the relationship between yoga and the nervous system, practitioners can tailor their practice to support nervous system health, manage stress more effectively, and achieve a state of balanced well-being. Integrating these practices into daily life not only enhances physical health but also fosters mental clarity, emotional resilience, and a deeper sense of inner peace.

CHAPTER 5

The Role of Breath (Pranayama) in Yoga Anatomy

Pranayama, the practice of breath control in yoga, is a cornerstone of yoga anatomy, as it directly influences the physiological and energetic systems of the body. "Prana" refers to the vital life force or energy, and "yama" means control or regulation. Through pranayama, practitioners can harness and direct this vital energy, promoting physical health, mental clarity, and spiritual growth.

Understanding Pranayama

Pranayama is more than just breathing exercises; it involves the conscious regulation of breath to influence the body and mind. Different pranayama techniques focus on various aspects of the breath, such as the rhythm, depth, and duration of inhalation, exhalation, and retention. These techniques are designed to enhance the flow of prana throughout the body, supporting overall well-being.

Anatomy of Breath

To fully understand the role of pranayama in yoga anatomy, it's important to explore the anatomical structures involved in breathing:

The Respiratory System

Lungs: The primary organs of respiration, the lungs are responsible for gas exchange, bringing oxygen into the body and expelling carbon dioxide.

Diaphragm: A dome-shaped muscle at the base of the lungs, the diaphragm is the primary muscle involved in breathing. During inhalation, the diaphragm contracts and moves downward, creating space for the lungs to expand. During exhalation, it relaxes and moves upward, helping to expel air from the lungs.

Intercostal Muscles: These muscles are located between the ribs and assist in the expansion and contraction of the chest cavity during breathing.

Accessory Muscles: Muscles such as the sternocleidomastoid, scalene, and pectoralis minor assist in deeper or labored breathing, particularly during physical exertion or in specific pranayama practices.

The Nervous System

Autonomic Nervous System (ANS): The ANS regulates involuntary bodily functions, including respiration. The practice of pranayama can influence the balance between the sympathetic (SNS) and parasympathetic (PNS) branches of the ANS, promoting either activation or relaxation depending on the technique used.

The Circulatory System

Blood Vessels: The circulatory system works closely with the respiratory system to transport oxygen-rich blood from the lungs to the rest of the body and return carbon dioxide-laden blood to the lungs for exhalation.

Heart Rate: Pranayama can affect heart rate by either increasing or decreasing it, depending on the breath pattern. Slow, deep breathing typically reduces heart rate and promotes relaxation, while rapid breathing can increase heart rate and stimulate the body.

Key Pranayama Techniques and Their Effects

Different pranayama techniques target various aspects of the respiratory system and have specific effects on the body and mind. Here are some key pranayama practices and their anatomical and physiological impacts:

Ujjayi Pranayama (Victorious Breath)

Technique: Ujjayi involves a gentle constriction of the throat (glottis) during both inhalation and exhalation, producing a soft, ocean-like sound.

Anatomical Impact: This practice increases the duration of each breath, encouraging deeper breathing and enhancing oxygenation of the blood. The constriction of the throat also engages the parasympathetic nervous system, promoting relaxation and focus.

Physiological Benefits: Ujjayi Pranayama helps calm the mind, reduce stress, and improve concentration. It is often used during asana practice to maintain a steady flow of breath and energy.
Nadi Shodhana (Alternate Nostril Breathing)

Technique: Nadi Shodhana involves alternating the breath between the left and right nostrils, using the fingers to close off one nostril at a time. This practice is typically slow and controlled, with equal duration for inhalation and exhalation.

Anatomical Impact: Nadi Shodhana balances the flow of air and prana through the nasal passages, which are connected to different branches of the autonomic nervous system. The right nostril is linked to the sympathetic nervous system (stimulating), and the left nostril to the parasympathetic nervous system (calming).

Physiological Benefits: This technique helps balance the nervous system, reduce stress, and promote mental clarity. It is particularly effective for calming the mind and preparing for meditation.

Kapalabhati (Skull Shining Breath)
Technique: Kapalabhati involves short, forceful exhalations followed by passive inhalations. The

diaphragm and abdominal muscles work vigorously to expel air from the lungs, while inhalations occur naturally without effort.

Anatomical Impact: Kapalabhati strengthens the diaphragm and abdominal muscles, enhances lung capacity, and stimulates the sympathetic nervous system. It also increases blood flow and oxygenation to the brain.

Physiological Benefits: This energizing practice helps clear the mind, invigorate the body, and improve focus. It is often used as a preparation for more intense physical or mental activity.

Bhramari (Bee Breath)

Technique: Bhramari involves inhaling deeply through the nose and exhaling while making a humming sound, similar to the sound of a bee. The sound is created by partially closing the glottis and allowing the vocal cords to vibrate during exhalation.

Anatomical Impact: The vibrations produced during Bhramari stimulate the vagus nerve, which activates the parasympathetic nervous system and promotes relaxation. The practice also helps to release tension in the throat and facial muscles.

Physiological Benefits: Bhramari Pranayama is effective for reducing anxiety, calming the mind, and improving concentration. The vibrations help to soothe the nervous system and create a sense of inner peace.

Sitali Pranayama (Cooling Breath)
Technique: Sitali involves inhaling through a curled tongue or pursed lips, which cools the air as it enters the body, followed by a slow exhalation through the nose.

Anatomical Impact: The cooling effect of the breath helps to lower body temperature, soothe the nervous system, and promote relaxation. This practice also engages the parasympathetic nervous system, encouraging a state of calm.

Physiological Benefits: Sitali Pranayama is particularly beneficial for reducing heat-related stress, calming the mind, and balancing the body's internal temperature. It is often practiced in hot weather or after vigorous physical activity.

Pranayama and the Mind-Body Connection
Pranayama is a powerful tool for cultivating the mind-body connection, as it requires conscious awareness of the breath and its effects on the body. By focusing on the breath, practitioners can bring their attention inward, fostering a deeper sense of mindfulness and presence. This connection between breath, body, and mind is central to the practice of yoga and has several key benefits:

Stress Reduction: Pranayama helps to regulate the nervous system, reducing the production of stress hormones and promoting relaxation. This leads to a decrease in anxiety, improved mood, and a greater sense of overall well-being.

Emotional Regulation: By consciously controlling the breath, practitioners can influence their emotional state. For example, deep, slow breathing can help to calm feelings of anger or frustration, while energizing breath practices can lift feelings of fatigue or depression.

Enhanced Focus and Concentration: Pranayama practices that involve breath retention (kumbhaka) or alternate nostril breathing can improve mental clarity and focus. These techniques help to quiet the mind, making it easier to concentrate on tasks or enter a meditative state.

Improved Physical Health: Regular pranayama practice can enhance respiratory function, increase lung capacity, and improve circulation. It also supports the body's natural detoxification processes by encouraging the release of carbon dioxide and other waste products from the lungs.

Spiritual Growth: In the broader context of yoga, pranayama is considered a gateway to higher states of consciousness. By mastering the breath, practitioners can control the flow of prana within the body, leading to deeper meditation and spiritual insight.

Integrating Pranayama into Your Yoga Practice
To fully experience the benefits of pranayama, it's important to integrate breath control into your regular yoga practice. Here are some tips for doing so:

Start with Awareness: Begin by simply observing your natural breath without trying to change it. Notice the rhythm, depth, and quality of your breath, and how it relates to your physical and emotional state.

Incorporate Pranayama Techniques: Gradually introduce specific pranayama techniques into your practice, starting with simple exercises like Ujjayi or Nadi Shodhana. Practice these techniques regularly, paying attention to how they affect your body and mind.

Use the Breath to Support Asana Practice: Coordinate your breath with movement during asana practice. For example, inhale as you extend or lift the body, and exhale as you fold or contract. This helps to create a sense of flow and balance in your practice.

Practice Pranayama in Stillness: Dedicate time to practicing pranayama in a seated or reclining position, without the distraction of movement. This allows you to fully focus on the breath and its effects on your body and mind.

Listen to Your Body: Pranayama should be practiced with care and respect for your body's limits. If you experience dizziness, shortness of breath, or discomfort, ease off the practice and return to a natural breath.

By embracing the practice of pranayama, you can unlock the full potential of your breath, enhancing your physical health, mental clarity, and spiritual well-being. Whether you are new to yoga or an experienced practitioner, pranayama offers a powerful way to deepen your connection to yourself and the world around you.

CHAPTER 6

Alignment Principles in Yoga

Alignment in yoga refers to the precise way in which the body should be positioned in each posture (asana) to ensure safety, effectiveness, and a deeper connection between the mind and body. Proper alignment helps to distribute the physical load evenly across muscles and joints, prevents injury, and allows for a more profound experience of the asanas.

Understanding and applying alignment principles is essential for both beginners and experienced practitioners. While alignment may vary depending on an individual's body structure, flexibility, and strength, certain fundamental principles apply to all yoga practices.

Key Alignment Principles in Yoga
Foundation and Grounding

Concept: The foundation of a pose refers to the parts of the body that are in contact with the ground. Proper grounding ensures stability and balance in the posture.

Application: In standing poses like Mountain Pose (Tadasana), the feet should be firmly rooted into the ground, with equal weight distributed across the heels, balls of the feet, and the outer edges. In seated poses, the sit bones should be evenly grounded to create a stable base.

Benefits: Grounding enhances balance, stability, and the flow of energy (prana) through the body. It also helps in building a strong connection between the body and the earth, providing a sense of stability and support.

Spinal Alignment
Concept: The spine is the central axis of the body, and its alignment is crucial for overall health and well-being. Proper spinal alignment maintains the natural curves of the spine—cervical (neck), thoracic (upper back), and lumbar (lower back)—and prevents strain or injury.

Application: In poses like Downward-Facing Dog (Adho Mukha Svanasana) or Cobra Pose (Bhujangasana), the spine should be elongated, with the head and neck in line with the rest of the spine. Avoid excessive rounding or arching of the back unless specifically required by the pose.

Benefits: Proper spinal alignment reduces the risk of back pain and injury, enhances posture, and allows for the free flow of energy along the spine. It also supports the respiratory system by maintaining an open and spacious chest.

Joint Alignment

Concept: Joint alignment involves positioning the joints in a way that distributes weight evenly and avoids hyperextension or compression. This principle is essential for protecting the joints, particularly in weight-bearing poses.

Application: In poses like Plank (Phalakasana) or Warrior II (Virabhadrasana II), ensure that the joints are stacked correctly. For example, the wrists should be aligned directly under the shoulders in Plank, and the knee should be directly over the ankle in Warrior II. Avoid locking the joints or placing them in positions that create undue stress.

Benefits: Proper joint alignment prevents strain, injury, and wear on the joints. It also promotes strength and stability in the muscles surrounding the joints, supporting overall joint health.

Engagement and Relaxation of Muscles
Concept: Effective alignment involves the active engagement of certain muscle groups while allowing others to relax. This balance of effort and ease (sthira and sukha) is a core principle of yoga.

Application: In poses like Tree Pose (Vrksasana), engage the core muscles to maintain balance, while allowing the shoulders and face to relax. In forward bends like Seated Forward Bend (Paschimottanasana), engage the thighs to protect the hamstrings, while releasing tension in the neck and shoulders.

Benefits: Balancing muscle engagement and relaxation prevents overexertion and injury, while promoting strength, flexibility, and a sense of ease in the practice. It also fosters mindfulness and awareness of the body.

Symmetry and Balance
Concept: Symmetry in yoga refers to maintaining evenness and balance between the right and left sides of the body, as well as between the front and back. This principle is important for creating harmony and preventing imbalances that could lead to injury.

Application: In poses like Triangle (Trikonasana), focus on aligning the right and left sides of the body evenly. In balancing poses like Tree Pose (Vrksasana), aim to distribute weight evenly between both feet or both sides of the body. Practice poses on both sides to maintain symmetry.

Benefits: Symmetry and balance in alignment promote equal development of strength and flexibility on both sides of the body. They also enhance proprioception (body awareness) and prevent compensatory patterns that can lead to imbalances.

Breath and Alignment

Concept: The breath is closely linked to alignment, as it provides feedback on the state of the body and helps to create space within the poses. Proper alignment should allow for smooth, unrestricted breathing.

Application: In poses like Bridge Pose (Setu Bandhasana) or Child's Pose (Balasana), align the body in a way that supports deep, even breathing. Avoid compressing the chest or abdomen in a way that restricts breath flow. Use the breath to guide and deepen the alignment in each pose.

Benefits: Synchronizing breath with alignment enhances relaxation, focus, and the flow of energy in the body. It also supports the parasympathetic nervous system, promoting a sense of calm and well-being during the practice.

Mindful Transitions

Concept: Alignment principles extend beyond static poses to the transitions between them. Moving mindfully between poses helps maintain alignment and prevents injury.

Application: When moving from Downward-Facing Dog (Adho Mukha Svanasana) to Plank (Phalakasana), for example, engage the core and move with control, maintaining the alignment of the shoulders, spine, and hips. Avoid rushing through transitions, as this can lead to misalignment and strain.

Benefits: Mindful transitions maintain the integrity of alignment throughout the practice, reducing the risk of injury. They also enhance the flow and rhythm of the practice, fostering a meditative and focused experience.

Individual Variations and Modifications
Concept: Every body is unique, and alignment should be adapted to suit individual needs, limitations, and abilities. This principle acknowledges that there is no one-size-fits-all approach to alignment.

Application: Use props like blocks, straps, or blankets to support proper alignment in poses. For example, in Triangle Pose (Trikonasana), use a block under the hand if reaching the floor compromises the alignment of the spine. Modify poses to accommodate injuries or limitations, such as bending the knees in Forward Folds (Uttanasana) to protect tight hamstrings.

Benefits: Adapting alignment to individual needs prevents injury, supports healing, and makes yoga accessible to everyone. It also fosters a sense of self-compassion and awareness of one's own body.

Applying Alignment Principles in Practice

To effectively apply these alignment principles in your yoga practice, consider the following tips:

Seek Guidance: Especially for beginners, working with a knowledgeable teacher who can provide personalized alignment cues is invaluable. They can help you understand your body's unique alignment needs and offer adjustments or modifications.

Use Props: Don't hesitate to use props like blocks, straps, and blankets to support your alignment. Props can help you achieve proper alignment and deepen your practice safely.

Practice Mindfulness: Pay close attention to your body's signals during practice. If you feel strain, discomfort, or restriction in your breath, it may indicate that your alignment needs adjustment.

Focus on the Fundamentals: Master the basics before attempting more advanced poses. Foundational poses like Mountain Pose (Tadasana), Downward-Facing Dog (Adho Mukha Svanasana), and Warrior I (Virabhadrasana I) provide essential alignment lessons that apply to more complex asanas.

Be Patient: Alignment takes time to develop, especially as you become more aware of your body's patterns and imbalances. Approach your practice with patience, and celebrate small improvements.

Listen to Your Body: Alignment is not about forcing your body into a perfect shape. Instead, it's about finding the version of the pose that best serves your body's needs in each moment. Always prioritize safety and comfort over aesthetics.

By understanding and applying alignment principles, you can deepen your yoga practice, prevent injury, and cultivate a greater awareness of your body. Whether you're a beginner or an experienced practitioner, these principles serve as a foundation for a safe, effective, and enriching yoga journey.

CHAPTER 7

Yoga Poses and Their Anatomical Focus

Yoga poses (asanas) are designed to work on specific areas of the body, targeting different muscles, joints, and organs. Each pose has a unique anatomical focus, offering various physical and mental benefits. Understanding the anatomical focus of each pose can help you tailor your practice to your individual needs, whether you aim to build strength, increase flexibility, improve balance, or enhance overall well-being.

Below is an overview of some common yoga poses categorized by their primary anatomical focus.

Standing Poses

Standing poses are foundational in yoga and work on building strength, stability, and balance. They primarily target the lower body, including the legs, hips, and core.

Mountain Pose (Tadasana)

Anatomical Focus: Entire body, with emphasis on alignment, posture, and grounding. Engages the thighs, calves, core, and muscles along the spine.
Benefits: Improves posture, strengthens legs and core, enhances body awareness.

Warrior I (Virabhadrasana I)

Anatomical Focus: Hips, thighs, calves, shoulders, and chest.
Benefits: Strengthens the legs and shoulders, opens the chest and hips, improves balance.

Warrior II (Virabhadrasana II)
Anatomical Focus: Hips, thighs, knees, ankles, and shoulders.
Benefits: Strengthens and stretches the legs and ankles, improves concentration, increases stamina.

Triangle Pose (Trikonasana)
Anatomical Focus: Hamstrings, hips, chest, shoulders, and spine.
Benefits: Stretches the legs, hips, and groin, opens the chest, improves flexibility in the spine.

Chair Pose (Utkatasana)
Anatomical Focus: Thighs, calves, spine, and shoulders.
Benefits: Strengthens the legs, glutes, and core, enhances stability, and builds endurance.

Forward Bends
Forward bends focus on stretching the posterior chain of the body, including the hamstrings, calves, and lower back. They also promote relaxation and stress relief.

Standing Forward Bend (Uttanasana)

Anatomical Focus: Hamstrings, calves, spine, and lower back.
Benefits: Stretches the hamstrings and calves, relieves tension in the spine, calms the mind.

Seated Forward Bend (Paschimottanasana)

Anatomical Focus: Hamstrings, calves, spine, and lower back.
Benefits: Stretches the entire back of the body, promotes relaxation, improves digestion.

Wide-Legged Forward Bend (Prasarita Padottanasana)

Anatomical Focus: Hamstrings, calves, spine, and hips.
Benefits: Stretches the inner thighs, hamstrings, and spine, strengthens the legs, calms the nervous system.

Backbends

Backbends focus on opening the front of the body, including the chest, shoulders, and abdomen. They strengthen the back muscles and improve spinal flexibility.

Cobra Pose (Bhujangasana)

Anatomical Focus: Spine, chest, shoulders, and lower back.
Benefits: Strengthens the spine, opens the chest and shoulders, improves posture.

Bridge Pose (Setu Bandhasana)

Anatomical Focus: Spine, hips, glutes, and thighs.
Benefits: Strengthens the back, glutes, and hamstrings, opens the chest, stretches the neck and spine.

Camel Pose (Ustrasana)

Anatomical Focus: Spine, chest, shoulders, and hips.
Benefits: Deeply opens the chest and shoulders, stretches the front of the body, strengthens the back muscles.

Upward-Facing Dog (Urdhva Mukha Svanasana)

Anatomical Focus: Spine, chest, shoulders, and arms.
Benefits: Opens the chest and shoulders, strengthens the arms and spine, improves posture.

Twists

Twisting poses target the spine and abdominal muscles, promoting detoxification and improving digestion. They also increase spinal mobility.

Revolved Triangle Pose (Parivrtta Trikonasana)

Anatomical Focus: Spine, hips, hamstrings, and shoulders.
Benefits: Stretches and strengthens the legs, improves digestion, increases spinal flexibility.
Half Lord of the Fishes Pose (Ardha Matsyendrasana)

Anatomical Focus: Spine, hips, and shoulders.
Benefits: Stretches the spine, hips, and shoulders, stimulates digestion, relieves lower back pain.

Seated Spinal Twist (Marichyasana)

Anatomical Focus: Spine, shoulders, and abdomen.
Benefits: Increases spinal flexibility, massages the abdominal organs, relieves tension in the back.

Balancing Poses

Balancing poses focus on stabilizing the core and improving proprioception (body awareness). They often engage multiple muscle groups and require concentration and mental focus.

Tree Pose (Vrksasana)

Anatomical Focus: Hips, thighs, calves, and core.
Benefits: Improves balance and stability, strengthens the legs, enhances concentration.

Eagle Pose (Garudasana)

Anatomical Focus: Shoulders, hips, thighs, calves, and core.
Benefits: Strengthens and stretches the ankles and calves, improves focus and balance, opens the shoulders and hips.

Crow Pose (Bakasana)

Anatomical Focus: Arms, wrists, core, and shoulders.

Benefits: Strengthens the arms and core, improves balance and focus, builds confidence.

Hip Openers

Hip openers focus on stretching and strengthening the muscles around the hips, including the hip flexors, glutes, and inner thighs. These poses help release tension and improve flexibility in the hips.

Pigeon Pose (Eka Pada Rajakapotasana)

Anatomical Focus: Hips, glutes, and lower back.
Benefits: Deeply stretches the hip flexors and glutes, relieves tension in the lower back, improves hip flexibility.

Butterfly Pose (Baddha Konasana)

Anatomical Focus: Inner thighs, hips, and groin.
Benefits: Stretches the inner thighs and groin, improves flexibility in the hips, promotes relaxation.

Lizard Pose (Utthan Pristhasana)

Anatomical Focus: Hips, hamstrings, and quadriceps.
Benefits: Opens the hips, stretches the hamstrings and quadriceps, strengthens the legs.

Inversions

Inversions involve positioning the heart above the head, reversing the usual effects of gravity on the body. They focus on building strength, improving circulation, and enhancing mental clarity.

Headstand (Sirsasana)
Anatomical Focus: Shoulders, arms, core, and neck.
Benefits: Strengthens the shoulders, arms, and core, improves circulation, enhances concentration and mental clarity.

Shoulder Stand (Sarvangasana)
Anatomical Focus: Shoulders, neck, core, and legs.
Benefits: Strengthens the shoulders and core, improves circulation, calms the nervous system.

Legs-Up-the-Wall Pose (Viparita Karani)
Anatomical Focus: Legs, lower back, and spine.
Benefits: Relieves tension in the legs and lower back, improves circulation, promotes relaxation.

Restorative Poses
Restorative poses focus on relaxation and recovery, allowing the body to rest and rejuvenate. These poses are often held for extended periods with the support of props.

Child's Pose (Balasana)
Anatomical Focus: Spine, hips, and thighs.
Benefits: Gently stretches the spine, hips, and thighs, calms the mind, promotes relaxation.

Corpse Pose (Savasana)

Anatomical Focus: Entire body, particularly the nervous system.
Benefits: Promotes deep relaxation, reduces stress, allows the body to integrate the benefits of the practice.

Reclining Bound Angle Pose (Supta Baddha Konasana)
Anatomical Focus: Hips, inner thighs, and chest.
Benefits: Opens the hips and chest, promotes relaxation, relieves stress.

Applying Anatomical Focus in Practice
To make the most of your yoga practice, consider the following tips:
Identify Your Goals: Whether you want to build strength, improve flexibility, or relieve stress, choose poses that align with your goals and focus on the relevant anatomical areas.

Practice Mindfully: Pay attention to the sensations in your body as you move through each pose. This awareness will help you understand how each pose affects different parts of your body and how to adjust your alignment for maximum benefit.

Balance Your Practice: Incorporate a variety of poses that target different anatomical areas to create a balanced practice that supports overall health and well-being.

Listen to Your Body: Every body is different, and it's essential to listen to your body's needs and limitations. Modify poses as needed to suit your unique anatomy, and avoid pushing yourself into discomfort.

By understanding the anatomical focus of each yoga pose, you can create a more intentional and effective practice that supports your physical, mental, and emotional well-being.

CHAPTER 8

Injury Prevention and Rehabilitation in Yoga

Yoga is a powerful practice for enhancing physical health, mental well-being, and spiritual growth. However, like any physical activity, it carries the potential for injury if not practiced mindfully. Understanding how to prevent injuries and how yoga can be used for rehabilitation is crucial for a safe and sustainable practice.

This section will cover the principles of injury prevention in yoga, common yoga-related injuries, and how yoga can aid in rehabilitation.

Principles of Injury Prevention in Yoga
Practice Mindful Awareness

Concept: Being fully present and aware of your body's sensations during practice is key to injury prevention. Mindful awareness allows you to notice discomfort or strain before it leads to injury.

Application: Pay attention to how each pose feels in your body, avoiding movements that cause sharp pain or discomfort. Use the breath to guide your practice and to stay attuned to your body's signals.

Prioritize Proper Alignment

Concept: Proper alignment ensures that your body is in the safest and most effective position during each pose, reducing the risk of strain or injury.

Application: Work with a qualified teacher to understand the correct alignment for each pose. Use mirrors, props, and gentle adjustments to maintain alignment, especially in challenging poses.

Warm Up Thoroughly

Concept: Warming up prepares your muscles and joints for the more intense stretches and movements in your practice, reducing the risk of injury.

Application: Begin your practice with gentle movements like Cat-Cow (Marjaryasana-Bitilasana), Sun Salutations (Surya Namaskar), or dynamic stretches to increase circulation and flexibility before moving into deeper poses.

Listen to Your Body's Limits

Concept: Pushing your body beyond its limits can lead to injury. Recognizing and respecting your current physical capabilities is essential for a safe practice.

Application: Avoid forcing yourself into poses that feel too intense or beyond your current flexibility and strength. Use modifications and props to make poses accessible and comfortable for your body.

Avoid Overuse

Concept: Repeating the same poses or movements without adequate rest can lead to overuse injuries, particularly in the wrists, shoulders, knees, and lower back.

Application: Vary your practice to work different muscle groups and give overused areas time to recover. Incorporate restorative poses and rest days into your routine.

Use Props and Modifications

Concept: Props such as blocks, straps, blankets, and bolsters can help you achieve proper alignment and support your body in challenging poses.

Application: Use props to make poses more accessible, especially if you are recovering from an injury or have limited flexibility. Modify poses to suit your body's needs and limitations.

Practice with Qualified Guidance

Concept: Practicing under the guidance of a knowledgeable yoga instructor can help you learn correct techniques, avoid common mistakes, and receive personalized adjustments.

Application: Attend classes with certified instructors, particularly if you are new to yoga or are working with injuries. Consider private sessions for individualized attention.

Maintain a Balanced Practice

Concept: A well-rounded practice that includes a mix of strength, flexibility, balance, and relaxation poses helps prevent imbalances that can lead to injury.

Application: Incorporate a variety of poses that target different muscle groups and include both active and restorative practices in your routine.

Common Yoga-Related Injuries

Despite its many benefits, yoga can lead to certain injuries, particularly if practiced without proper alignment, awareness, or respect for the body's limits. Some common yoga-related injuries include:

Wrist Strain

Cause: Weight-bearing poses like Downward-Facing Dog (Adho Mukha Svanasana) or Plank (Phalakasana) can place strain on the wrists, especially if alignment is incorrect or if the wrists are weak.

Prevention: Distribute weight evenly across the hands, engage the forearms, and avoid locking the elbows. Use props or modifications to reduce wrist strain.

Lower Back Pain

Cause: Forward bends, twists, and backbends can cause lower back pain if performed with poor alignment or if the core is not engaged.

Prevention: Maintain a neutral spine, engage the core muscles, and avoid rounding the lower back in forward bends. Use props to support the back in challenging poses.

Hamstring Injuries

Cause: Overstretching in poses like Forward Bends (Uttanasana) or Triangle Pose (Trikonasana) can lead to hamstring strain or tears.

Prevention: Warm up thoroughly, engage the thigh muscles, and avoid forcing deep stretches. Use a slight bend in the knees if needed.

Shoulder Injuries

Cause: Incorrect alignment in poses like Chaturanga Dandasana, Downward-Facing Dog, or arm balances can strain the shoulder muscles and joints.

Prevention: Keep the shoulders engaged and aligned with the wrists, avoid sinking into the joints, and build shoulder strength gradually.

Knee Injuries

Cause: Misalignment in poses like Warrior I or II (Virabhadrasana I or II), or deep hip openers like Pigeon Pose (Eka Pada Rajakapotasana), can strain or injure the knees.

Prevention: Ensure the knees are aligned with the ankles, avoid twisting the knee joint, and use props to support the hips and knees.

Neck Strain

Cause: Strain in the neck can occur in poses like Headstand (Sirsasana), Shoulder Stand (Sarvangasana), or poses where the head is unsupported.

Prevention: Keep the neck long and in alignment with the spine, avoid excessive pressure on the cervical spine, and use props like blankets for support.

Yoga for Rehabilitation

Yoga is not only beneficial for injury prevention but also plays a significant role in rehabilitation. With its emphasis on gentle movement, breath awareness, and relaxation, yoga can aid in the recovery process for various injuries and conditions.

Restorative Yoga

Focus: Restorative yoga involves gentle, supported poses that promote relaxation and healing. It's particularly beneficial for recovery from injuries, surgery, or chronic conditions.

Application: Poses like Supported Child's Pose (Balasana), Reclining Bound Angle Pose (Supta Baddha Konasana), and Legs-Up-the-Wall Pose (Viparita Karani) can help reduce pain, improve circulation, and promote relaxation.

Therapeutic Yoga

Focus: Therapeutic yoga is tailored to the individual's specific needs and conditions, using poses, breathwork, and meditation to support healing.

Application: Work with a certified yoga therapist to develop a personalized practice that addresses your specific injury or condition. Therapeutic yoga can help with conditions like back pain, arthritis, or post-surgery recovery.

Strengthening and Stabilization

Focus: Yoga can help rebuild strength and stability in muscles and joints after an injury. Focus on poses that target the affected area, gradually increasing intensity as healing progresses.

Application: Poses like Bridge Pose (Setu Bandhasana), Warrior I and II (Virabhadrasana I and II), and Plank (Phalakasana) can strengthen the core, legs, and back, supporting injury recovery.

Flexibility and Mobility

Focus: Gentle stretching and mobility exercises can help restore flexibility and range of motion after an injury. Yoga poses that focus on lengthening and opening the muscles can aid in this process.

Application: Poses like Cat-Cow (Marjaryasana-Bitilasana), Gentle Twists (Supta Matsyendrasana), and Reclined Hand-to-Big-Toe Pose (Supta Padangusthasana) can help restore flexibility without overstretching.

Breathwork (Pranayama)

Focus: Breathwork can support the healing process by reducing stress, improving circulation, and enhancing relaxation. Deep, mindful breathing can also help manage pain.

Application: Practice gentle pranayama techniques like Diaphragmatic Breathing, Nadi Shodhana (Alternate Nostril Breathing), and Ujjayi Breath to support recovery and relaxation.

Mindfulness and Stress Reduction

Focus: Yoga's emphasis on mindfulness and meditation can help manage the emotional and psychological aspects of injury recovery. Stress reduction is a crucial component of the healing process.

Application: Incorporate mindfulness practices like Body Scan Meditation, Loving-Kindness Meditation, or simple breath awareness into your yoga practice to reduce stress and promote healing.

Tips for Safe Rehabilitation with Yoga

Consult with Healthcare Providers: Before starting or continuing a yoga practice during injury recovery, consult with your healthcare provider, physical therapist, or a certified yoga therapist to ensure that the poses and movements are safe for your specific condition.

Start Slow and Gentle: Begin with gentle movements and simple poses that do not exacerbate your injury. Gradually increase the intensity and duration of your practice as your body heals.

Use Props and Modifications: Props like blocks, straps, and bolsters can support your body in poses, making them more accessible and comfortable. Modify poses as needed to avoid strain.

Listen to Your Body: Pay close attention to your body's signals. If a pose causes pain or discomfort, back off or modify it. Avoid pushing yourself into poses that feel too intense.

Be Patient: Healing takes time, and it's essential to be patient with your body's recovery process. Focus on gentle, consistent practice rather than pushing for quick results.

Incorporate Restorative Practices: Include restorative yoga, pranayama, and meditation in your practice to support the healing process and promote relaxation.

By practicing yoga mindfully and incorporating injury prevention and rehabilitation principles, you can enjoy the many benefits of yoga while minimizing the risk of injury and supporting your body's recovery process.

CHAPTER 9

Integrating Anatomy into Yoga Practice

Understanding anatomy is essential for deepening your yoga practice, ensuring safety, and maximizing the benefits of each pose. By integrating anatomical knowledge into your practice, you can enhance alignment, prevent injuries, and tailor your practice to your body's unique needs. This section explores how to effectively incorporate anatomical principles into your yoga routine.

Understanding Body Mechanics in Yoga

Body mechanics refers to how the body moves and functions in various poses. Understanding body mechanics helps you move more efficiently, maintain proper alignment, and reduce the risk of injury.

Alignment Awareness: Knowing the anatomical landmarks and natural curves of the spine (cervical, thoracic, lumbar) helps you maintain proper alignment in poses like Mountain Pose (Tadasana) or Downward-Facing Dog (Adho Mukha Svanasana). Aligning the joints—shoulders, hips, knees, and ankles—ensures that the body's weight is distributed evenly, reducing strain.

Movement Patterns: Understanding the different types of movement—flexion, extension, rotation, abduction, adduction—allows you to explore the full range of motion in your joints safely. For example, in a forward fold (Uttanasana), knowing that the movement involves hip flexion with a straight spine helps you avoid rounding the lower back.

Applying Anatomical Principles to Poses

Each yoga pose targets specific muscles, joints, and connective tissues. Applying anatomical principles can help you engage the right muscles and protect vulnerable areas.

Muscle Engagement: Engaging the correct muscles helps stabilize the body in challenging poses. For example, in Warrior II (Virabhadrasana II), engaging the quadriceps and glutes supports the knees and prevents overextension.

Joint Protection: Understanding the structure of joints helps you avoid hyperextension or misalignment. In poses like Plank (Phalakasana), maintaining a slight bend in the elbows protects the delicate structures of the elbow joint.

Breath and Movement: Coordinating breath with movement supports the nervous system and enhances focus. For instance, inhaling during a backbend (like Cobra Pose) expands the chest and supports the spine, while exhaling in a forward fold allows for deeper relaxation and stretching.

Tailoring Your Practice to Your Anatomy

Each person's anatomy is unique, and recognizing this individuality can help you tailor your practice to suit your body's specific needs.

Personalized Modifications: Understanding your body's strengths and limitations allows you to modify poses for safety and comfort. For instance, if you have tight hamstrings, using a block in a forward fold can prevent strain on the lower back.

Injury Consideration: If you have a history of injuries, such as a knee or shoulder injury, anatomical knowledge enables you to adjust your practice to avoid aggravating those areas. This might involve avoiding deep knee bends or modifying arm balances to reduce pressure on the shoulder joint.

Props for Support: Using props like blocks, straps, and bolsters helps accommodate different body types and flexibility levels. Props can also assist in maintaining alignment, such as placing a block under the sacrum in Bridge Pose (Setu Bandhasana) for added support.

Enhancing Mind-Body Awareness

Integrating anatomy into yoga enhances mind-body awareness—the ability to connect with and understand the body's internal signals and alignment.

Proprioception: Proprioception is the body's ability to sense its position in space. Enhanced proprioception allows for better alignment and balance in poses. For example, focusing on grounding through the feet in Tree Pose (Vrksasana) improves stability and alignment.

Body Scanning: Regularly scanning the body during practice helps identify areas of tension or misalignment. This practice encourages you to make subtle adjustments to improve comfort and effectiveness in each pose.

Mindful Movement: Moving mindfully, with an awareness of how each part of the body engages, reduces the risk of injury and increases the effectiveness of the pose. Mindful movement also connects the physical practice of yoga with its meditative aspects.

Using Anatomy for Injury Prevention
Anatomy plays a crucial role in injury prevention by helping you understand how to move safely and avoid common pitfalls.

Avoiding Overstretching: Knowing the limits of your muscles and connective tissues prevents overstretching, which can lead to strains or tears. In poses like Forward Bend (Paschimottanasana), gently easing into the stretch rather than forcing it helps protect the hamstrings.

Balanced Practice: A well-rounded practice that includes strengthening, stretching, and balancing poses supports overall joint health and reduces the likelihood of overuse injuries. For example, balancing backbends with forward bends helps maintain spinal health and flexibility.

Safe Transitions: Moving safely between poses is as important as the poses themselves. Understanding the anatomical implications of transitions, such as moving from Downward-Facing Dog to Plank, ensures that you protect the wrists, shoulders, and lower back.

Teaching with Anatomical Awareness
For yoga teachers, integrating anatomy into teaching enhances the ability to guide students safely and effectively.

Cueing Alignment: Using anatomical cues helps students understand how to position their bodies correctly. For example, instructing students to "draw the shoulder blades down the back" in Cobra Pose (Bhujangasana) promotes proper shoulder alignment.

Addressing Individual Needs: Being aware of different body types and anatomical variations allows teachers to offer personalized adjustments and modifications. This might involve suggesting a prop or offering an alternative pose to accommodate a student's unique anatomy.

Promoting Safe Practice: Teaching students about the anatomy involved in each pose empowers them to practice more safely and confidently, reducing the risk of injury and enhancing their overall experience.

Integrating anatomy into your yoga practice offers numerous benefits, from improving alignment and preventing injuries to deepening your mind-body connection. By understanding the mechanics of your body, you can practice yoga with greater awareness, safety, and effectiveness. Whether you're a practitioner seeking to enhance your practice or a teacher aiming to guide others, incorporating anatomical principles is essential for a holistic and sustainable yoga journey.

CHAPTER 10

Advanced Yoga Anatomy

Advanced yoga anatomy delves deeper into the intricate details of how the body functions during complex yoga poses and practices. It involves a more nuanced understanding of anatomy, including the interactions between different body systems, detailed muscle functions, and the impact of advanced asanas on the body. This knowledge enhances your ability to practice and teach yoga safely and effectively, particularly in advanced poses and sequences.

Advanced Muscular Function and Interaction
Muscle Synergies:

Concept: Advanced yoga poses often require multiple muscle groups to work together in complex ways. Understanding muscle synergies—how muscles collaborate to produce movement—can enhance your practice and teaching.

Application: In poses like Handstand (Adho Mukha Vrksasana), the core, shoulders, and arms work synergistically. Knowing which muscles engage and how they support each other helps in fine-tuning alignment and strength.

Deep Core Muscles:

Concept: Beyond the superficial abdominal muscles (rectus abdominis), the deep core muscles

(transverse abdominis, multifidus, pelvic floor) play a crucial role in stabilizing the spine and pelvis.
Application: Strengthening these deep core muscles supports advanced poses such as Arm Balances (Bakasana), where core stability is essential. Incorporate exercises that target these muscles, like abdominal draws or pelvic floor engagement.

Complex Joint Mechanics
Hip Joint Mobility and Stability:
Concept: The hip joint's range of motion and stability are vital for advanced poses that require deep external and internal rotation, such as Pigeon Pose (Eka Pada Rajakapotasana).
Application: Understanding the anatomy of the hip joint and its surrounding muscles helps in safely performing deep hip openers and preventing injuries. Work on both flexibility and strength around the hip joint for balanced mobility.

Shoulder Joint Dynamics:
Concept: The shoulder joint is highly mobile and relies on the stability of surrounding muscles, including the rotator cuff. Advanced poses like Handstand (Adho Mukha Vrksasana) and Crow Pose (Bakasana) require intricate shoulder mechanics.
Application: Strengthen and stabilize the rotator cuff muscles and practice proper alignment to prevent shoulder injuries. Incorporate shoulder stability

exercises and be mindful of shoulder positioning in weight-bearing poses.

Advanced Spinal Movements
Spinal Flexibility and Extension:
Concept: Advanced yoga poses often involve significant spinal flexion (e.g., Forward Folds), extension (e.g., Backbends), and rotation (e.g., Twists). Understanding the anatomy of spinal segments and intervertebral discs is crucial.
Application: Practice advanced poses with awareness of spinal alignment and range of motion. Use modifications and props as needed to ensure safe and effective spinal movement, particularly in deep backbends or twists.

Segmental Movement:
Concept: The spine is divided into different segments (cervical, thoracic, lumbar, sacral). Each segment moves differently, and understanding these differences helps in maintaining proper alignment.
Application: In poses like Wheel Pose (Urdhva Dhanurasana), engage and stretch each spinal segment appropriately. Awareness of segmental movement helps in achieving a balanced and safe practice.

Advanced Anatomical Considerations in Poses
Handstands and Arm Balances:

Concept: These poses require complex interactions between the shoulders, core, and wrists. Understanding the detailed anatomy of these areas helps in building strength and stability.
Application: Strengthen the shoulders, core, and wrists through targeted exercises. Focus on alignment and engagement in poses like Handstand (Adho Mukha Vrksasana) to ensure safety and effectiveness.
Inversions and Blood Flow:

Concept: Inversions change the body's orientation and impact blood flow and pressure. Understanding how these poses affect the cardiovascular system is important for safety.
Application: Be mindful of blood flow and pressure changes in poses like Headstand (Sirsasana) and Shoulder Stand (Sarvangasana). Ensure proper alignment and use props to support the body in inversions.

Advanced Respiratory Mechanics
Pranayama and Advanced Poses:
Concept: Advanced pranayama techniques and poses require an understanding of the respiratory system and how breath affects the body's mechanics.
Application: Practice advanced pranayama techniques, such as Kapalabhati or Bhastrika, in conjunction with complex poses. Understand how

breath control influences muscle engagement and relaxation.

Diaphragm and Core Integration:
Concept: The diaphragm plays a key role in both respiration and core stability. Advanced poses often require coordinated diaphragm function and core engagement.
Application: Integrate breath awareness with core strengthening exercises. Practice poses like Leg Lifts (Uttanapadasana) or Boat Pose (Navasana) while focusing on diaphragmatic breathing.

Advanced Anatomy in Teaching
Detailed Cueing:
Concept: Advanced anatomical knowledge allows for precise and detailed cueing in teaching. This enhances students' understanding and execution of complex poses.
Application: Use anatomical terminology and detailed cues to guide students in advanced poses. For example, in a complex balance pose, instruct students to engage specific muscles or align joints accurately.

Customized Adjustments:
Concept: Advanced anatomical insights enable you to provide customized adjustments based on individual students' anatomical variations and needs.
Application: Observe students' body mechanics and offer personalized adjustments. For instance,

provide support for students who struggle with shoulder stability in handstands.

Preventative and Rehabilitative Approaches:
Concept: Understanding advanced anatomy helps in designing practices that prevent injuries and support rehabilitation for students with specific needs.
Application: Create practices that address common issues related to advanced poses, such as shoulder stability or hip flexibility. Offer modifications and restorative options for students recovering from injuries.

Integrating Advanced Anatomy into Practice Self-Assessment:
Concept: Regularly assess your own body mechanics and alignment to ensure that you are practicing advanced poses safely and effectively.
Application: Use mirrors, videos, or feedback from teachers to evaluate and adjust your alignment and technique in advanced poses.

Continual Learning:
Concept: Anatomy is a dynamic field, and ongoing education enhances your understanding and application of advanced anatomical principles.
Application: Stay updated with new anatomical research, attend advanced workshops, and consult with experts to deepen your anatomical knowledge and improve your practice.

Mind-Body Connection:
Concept: Advanced anatomy is not just about physical understanding but also about integrating this knowledge with the mind-body connection.

Application: Use anatomical insights to enhance your awareness of how the body moves and feels in advanced poses. Combine this understanding with mindful practice to achieve a balanced and effective yoga experience.

By integrating advanced anatomy into your yoga practice, you can deepen your understanding of body mechanics, enhance the effectiveness of complex poses, and promote safety and well-being in both personal practice and teaching.

CHAPTER 11

Case Studies: Anatomical Insights in Yoga

Case studies offer practical examples of how anatomical insights are applied to address various challenges and enhance the practice of yoga. These case studies illustrate how understanding anatomy can lead to more effective and personalized yoga practices, injury prevention, and rehabilitation. Below are a few case studies highlighting different anatomical issues and their solutions through yoga practice.

Case Study: Improving Shoulder Stability in Handstands

Background:

A 35-year-old yoga practitioner, Sarah, experiences shoulder pain and instability while attempting Handstands (Adho Mukha Vrksasana). Despite regular practice, she struggles to maintain balance and experiences discomfort in the shoulder joints.

Anatomical Insight:

Shoulder instability often results from weakness or imbalances in the rotator cuff muscles and the surrounding shoulder girdle. Proper engagement and alignment of these muscles are crucial for stabilizing the shoulder joint during weight-bearing poses.

Solution:

Strengthening Exercises: Incorporate exercises to strengthen the rotator cuff muscles, such as external rotations with a resistance band and shoulder blade squeezes.

Alignment Cues: Focus on proper alignment in weight-bearing poses. Instruct Sarah to actively engage her shoulder blades by drawing them down and together, and to maintain a slight bend in the elbows to avoid hyperextension.

Modified Practice: Use wall support for Handstands to reduce pressure on the shoulders. Practice against a wall allows for adjustment and better alignment.

Outcome:

Sarah reports improved shoulder stability and reduced pain after incorporating strengthening exercises and alignment cues into her practice. She gains more confidence in performing Handstands with proper form.

Case Study: Managing Lower Back Pain in Forward Folds

Background:

John, a 45-year-old office worker, experiences lower back pain during Forward Folds (Uttanasana). His job involves long periods of sitting, which has led to tight hamstrings and lower back discomfort.

Anatomical Insight:

Lower back pain during Forward Folds can result from tight hamstrings and poor spinal alignment. The hamstrings' tightness can pull on the pelvis, causing the lower back to round and create strain.

Solution:
Hamstring Stretching: Introduce gentle hamstring stretches and strengthening exercises. Use props such as blocks under the hands in Forward Folds to modify the pose and reduce strain on the lower back.
Spinal Alignment: Emphasize maintaining a flat back and hinge from the hips rather than rounding the spine. Encourage John to keep a slight bend in the knees if needed.
Core Engagement: Strengthen the core muscles to support the lower back. Include exercises such as Boat Pose (Navasana) and Plank (Phalakasana) to build core stability.

Outcome:
John experiences reduced lower back pain and increased flexibility after incorporating hamstring stretches, proper alignment techniques, and core strengthening exercises into his practice.

Case Study: Enhancing Hip Flexibility for Pigeon Pose
Background:
Lisa, a 28-year-old yoga enthusiast, struggles with tight hips during Pigeon Pose (Eka Pada

Rajakapotasana). She experiences discomfort and limited range of motion, particularly on her right side.

Anatomical Insight:
Tight hips can result from shortened hip flexors, adductors, and external rotators. Understanding the anatomy of these muscles helps in addressing flexibility and discomfort.

Solution:
Targeted Stretching: Incorporate targeted hip stretches and mobility exercises, such as Hip Flexor Stretch (Lunge Pose) and Butterfly Pose (Baddha Konasana).
Use of Props: Use props like blocks or bolsters under the hips in Pigeon Pose to provide support and reduce strain.
Gradual Progression: Encourage a gradual approach to deepening the pose, using modifications and adjustments to accommodate Lisa's current flexibility.

Outcome:
Lisa notices improved hip flexibility and comfort in Pigeon Pose after consistently practicing targeted stretches and using props to support her hips.

Case Study: Rehabilitation of Wrist Injury with Yoga
Background:

Mark, a 32-year-old yoga teacher, sustains a wrist injury while practicing Chaturanga Dandasana (Four-Limbed Staff Pose). He experiences pain and limited mobility in the wrist.

Anatomical Insight:
Wrist injuries from yoga can result from improper weight distribution and overuse. Understanding the anatomy of the wrist joint and surrounding muscles helps in designing a rehabilitation plan.

Solution:
Rest and Recovery: Begin with a period of rest and avoid poses that place direct weight on the wrists.
Gentle Wrist Exercises: Incorporate gentle wrist exercises, such as wrist circles and stretches, to improve mobility and strength.
Modified Poses: Use modifications such as practicing on fists or forearms instead of hands to reduce stress on the wrists. Reinforce proper alignment and weight distribution in poses.

Outcome:
Mark's wrist injury improves with rest, modified poses, and targeted wrist exercises. He returns to full practice with increased awareness of wrist care and alignment.

Case Study: Addressing Neck Strain in Headstands
Background:

Emily, a 40-year-old advanced practitioner, experiences neck strain during Headstands (Sirsasana). She has a history of neck issues and wants to ensure her practice is safe.

Anatomical Insight:
Neck strain in Headstands can result from improper alignment or overloading the cervical spine. Understanding the anatomy of the cervical vertebrae and surrounding muscles is essential for safe practice.

Solution:
Strengthening and Alignment: Focus on strengthening the neck and upper back muscles. Practice supported Headstands with a cushion or blanket under the head to reduce strain.
Proper Technique: Ensure Emily's weight is distributed evenly between the head, forearms, and core. Avoid placing excessive weight on the neck and maintain a neutral spine.
Alternative Poses: Introduce alternative inversions or variations, such as Dolphin Pose (Ardha Pincha Mayurasana), to build strength and confidence while reducing neck strain.

Outcome:
Emily successfully integrates safer techniques and modifications into her practice, reducing neck strain and improving her overall experience in Headstands.

Case studies like these illustrate how anatomical insights can address various challenges in yoga practice. By understanding the specific anatomical issues related to different poses, practitioners and teachers can develop targeted solutions to enhance safety, effectiveness, and overall well-being. Whether dealing with common issues or advanced poses, integrating anatomical knowledge into yoga practice provides valuable tools for optimizing performance and preventing injuries.

CHAPTER 12

Conclusion

Yoga Anatomy is a vital aspect of both practicing and teaching yoga, offering profound insights into how the body moves, supports itself, and interacts during different poses. By understanding anatomy, you can significantly enhance your practice, prevent injuries, and achieve more effective and personalized results.

Key Takeaways:

Foundation of Knowledge: A solid grasp of anatomical principles—covering the muscular, skeletal, and connective tissue systems—provides a foundation for safe and effective yoga practice. It helps practitioners understand how different muscles and joints work together to support and challenge the body.

Injury Prevention: Awareness of anatomical insights aids in identifying potential risks and preventing injuries. Proper alignment, muscle engagement, and mindful modifications based on anatomical knowledge reduce the likelihood of strain and discomfort.

Personalization: Recognizing individual anatomical variations allows for a more tailored practice. Customizing poses and sequences to suit personal needs enhances comfort and effectiveness, supporting both beginners and advanced practitioners in their yoga journey.

Enhanced Practice: Integrating anatomical understanding into practice deepens the connection between mind and body. It helps practitioners engage muscles more consciously, align their bodies properly, and achieve greater flexibility, strength, and stability.

Teaching and Communication: For yoga teachers, anatomical knowledge improves the ability to guide students effectively. Detailed cueing, personalized adjustments, and injury prevention strategies enrich the teaching experience, promoting a safer and more supportive environment.

Continuous Learning: Anatomy is a dynamic field, and ongoing education is crucial for staying updated with new insights and practices. Continual learning enhances both personal practice and teaching, fostering a more informed and effective approach to yoga.

By integrating these anatomical insights into your yoga practice and teaching, you can cultivate a more mindful, safe, and effective practice, ensuring that both you and your students can enjoy the full benefits of yoga while minimizing risks.

The Future of Yoga Anatomy

As yoga continues to evolve and integrate with advancements in science and technology, the future of yoga anatomy promises to bring deeper insights, innovative practices, and enhanced safety. Here are several key trends and developments likely to shape the future of yoga anatomy:

Advancements in Technology and Research
Enhanced Imaging Techniques:

MRI and CT Scans: Advances in imaging technology, such as high-resolution MRI and CT scans, provide detailed views of muscle, joint, and connective tissue structures. These tools help in understanding the impact of various yoga poses on internal structures, leading to more precise and informed practice recommendations.

Functional Movement Analysis: Technologies like motion capture and 3D modeling offer insights into body mechanics during yoga practice. These tools can help in analyzing and optimizing movement patterns, improving alignment, and enhancing performance.

Wearable Technology:

Biofeedback Devices: Wearable devices that monitor muscle activity, heart rate, and posture can offer real-time feedback during yoga practice. These devices help practitioners understand their body's responses and adjust their practice for better alignment and effectiveness.

Virtual Reality (VR): VR technology can simulate yoga poses and movements, allowing practitioners to visualize and correct their alignment in a virtual environment. This can enhance learning and practice, particularly for complex poses.

Integrating Yoga with Modern Science
Evidence-Based Practices:
Research Integration: As scientific research on yoga anatomy and physiology grows, integrating evidence-based practices into yoga instruction can enhance safety and efficacy. Research studies on muscle engagement, joint health, and the effects of yoga on various conditions contribute to more effective and personalized practices.
Collaborative Studies: Collaboration between yoga practitioners and medical researchers can lead to a better understanding of how yoga influences health and well-being. This interdisciplinary approach can refine anatomical insights and support the development of best practices.

Personalized Medicine:
Genetics and Yoga: Advances in genetic research may offer insights into how individual genetic profiles affect flexibility, strength, and susceptibility to injuries. Personalized yoga programs tailored to genetic information could optimize practice and improve outcomes.
Biomarkers: The study of biomarkers related to yoga practice, such as stress hormones or inflammatory

markers, can provide insights into how yoga affects physiological processes. This information can help in designing practices that support specific health needs.

Evolving Yoga Practices
Functional Movement Integration:
Biomechanics: The integration of biomechanics into yoga practice enhances the understanding of how different body parts interact during movement. This approach helps in refining techniques and aligning poses to reduce strain and improve effectiveness.
Dynamic Movement: Emphasis on dynamic movement patterns and functional strength training complements traditional yoga practices. Incorporating these elements can address functional movement needs and enhance overall physical fitness.

Holistic Approaches:
Mind-Body Connection: Future developments in yoga anatomy will likely emphasize the integration of mind-body practices, including meditation, mindfulness, and emotional well-being. Understanding the anatomical basis of stress responses and relaxation can lead to more holistic and effective practices.
Integrative Therapies: Combining yoga with other therapeutic modalities, such as physical therapy or massage, can provide a comprehensive approach to injury prevention and rehabilitation. This integrative

approach enhances the effectiveness of yoga in supporting overall health.

Education and Training Innovations
Advanced Training Programs:
Specialized Courses: Future yoga teacher training programs may include more advanced anatomical courses, focusing on detailed knowledge of muscle function, joint mechanics, and injury prevention. Specialized training can help teachers offer more nuanced and effective instruction.
Online Learning Platforms: Online platforms offer opportunities for continuous learning and professional development in yoga anatomy. Virtual workshops, courses, and webinars can provide access to cutting-edge knowledge and techniques from anywhere in the world.

Collaborative Learning:
Interdisciplinary Collaboration: Collaborations between yoga practitioners, physiotherapists, and medical professionals can lead to more comprehensive and evidence-based anatomical education. This collaborative approach can enhance the quality of yoga training and instruction.

Accessibility and Inclusivity
Adaptive Yoga:
Inclusive Practices: Future advancements in yoga anatomy will likely focus on creating adaptive

practices that accommodate diverse body types, abilities, and needs. This includes developing modifications and props to make yoga accessible to everyone.

Trauma-Informed Yoga: Incorporating trauma-informed approaches into yoga practice acknowledges the impact of past experiences on the body. Understanding the anatomical and psychological aspects of trauma can lead to more supportive and healing practices.

Global Perspectives:
Cultural Integration: The future of yoga anatomy will benefit from integrating global perspectives and traditional knowledge with modern scientific understanding. This inclusive approach honors diverse yoga practices and enhances the richness of anatomical insights.

The future of yoga anatomy holds exciting possibilities, driven by technological advancements, scientific research, and a deeper understanding of the mind-body connection. By embracing these developments, yoga practitioners and teachers can continue to refine their practices, enhance safety, and support overall well-being. The integration of modern science with traditional practices will foster a more informed, inclusive, and effective approach to yoga, benefiting practitioners of all levels and backgrounds.

Continuing Education in Yoga and Anatomy
Continuing education in yoga and anatomy is essential for both practitioners and teachers to stay updated with the latest advancements, deepen their understanding, and enhance their practice and instruction. As the field of yoga evolves, ongoing learning ensures that individuals can offer safe, effective, and informed practices. Here's a comprehensive guide to continuing education in yoga and anatomy:

Specialized Courses and Workshops
Advanced Anatomy Courses:
Focus: These courses delve into detailed anatomical knowledge, including complex muscle interactions, joint mechanics, and the impact of advanced poses.
Providers: Look for workshops offered by reputable yoga schools, anatomy experts, or institutions specializing in yoga therapy and physical health.

Therapeutic Yoga Workshops:
Focus: Workshops that emphasize therapeutic applications of yoga, including injury prevention, rehabilitation, and working with specific conditions (e.g., back pain, hip issues).
Providers: Consider courses from yoga therapy organizations or healthcare professionals with expertise in yoga therapy.

Pranayama and Breath Work:

Focus: Advanced techniques and the anatomical basis of breath control (pranayama), including the impact on the respiratory system and overall health.
Providers: Workshops led by experienced pranayama instructors or institutions with a focus on breath-based practices.

Certification Programs
Yoga Teacher Training (YTT) Updates:
Focus: Continuing education programs that offer updates and advanced certifications in yoga teaching, incorporating new anatomical insights and teaching methodologies.
Providers: Reputable yoga schools and organizations that offer advanced YTT programs or specialized certifications (e.g., in alignment, anatomy, or therapeutic yoga).

Yoga Therapy Certification:
Focus: Certification programs for yoga therapists, emphasizing anatomical knowledge, therapeutic techniques, and working with specific health conditions.
Providers: Accredited yoga therapy institutions and professional organizations.

Online Learning Platforms
Webinars and Online Courses:
Focus: Accessible online courses and webinars covering various aspects of yoga anatomy, practice,

and teaching. Topics can range from basic anatomy to advanced biomechanical principles.
Providers: Platforms such as Yoga Alliance, Udemy, Coursera, and specialized yoga education websites.

Virtual Workshops and Conferences:
Focus: Participate in virtual workshops and conferences that provide opportunities for learning from experts, networking with other practitioners, and staying updated on the latest research.
Providers: Yoga associations, educational institutions, and professional organizations.

Books and Journals
Recommended Reading:
Focus: Stay updated with the latest publications on yoga anatomy, Including books by recognized experts in the field.
Examples: Books such as "Yoga Anatomy" by Leslie Kaminoff and "The Key Muscles of Yoga" by Ray Long provide detailed anatomical insights.

Academic Journals:
Focus: Read research articles and studies published in academic journals related to yoga, anatomy, and related fields.
Examples: Journals like the "Journal of Bodywork and Movement Therapies" or "International Journal of Yoga Therapy."

Practical Experience
Hands-On Practice:
Focus: Engage in practical experience by participating in workshops, working with anatomy experts, and applying new knowledge in your practice or teaching.
Providers: Look for workshops that offer hands-on practice with anatomical models, props, or personalized instruction.

Peer Learning and Practice Groups:
Focus: Join study groups or peer networks to discuss anatomical insights, share experiences, and collaborate on practice and teaching.
Providers: Yoga studios, professional networks, or online forums for yoga practitioners and teachers.

Collaboration and Networking
Professional Associations:
Focus: Join professional organizations and associations that offer resources, networking opportunities, and continuing education in yoga and anatomy.
Examples: Yoga Alliance, International Association of Yoga Therapists (IAYT), or local yoga associations.

Conferences and Seminars:
Focus: Attend conferences and seminars to learn from experts, explore new trends, and engage with the yoga community.

Examples: Annual yoga conferences, anatomy-focused seminars, or interdisciplinary events combining yoga and health sciences.

Integrating Knowledge into Practice
Applying New Insights:
Focus: Integrate new anatomical knowledge and techniques into your personal practice or teaching, adjusting poses and sequences based on updated information.
Examples: Incorporate advanced alignment techniques, new modifications, or therapeutic approaches into your classes.

Teaching Innovations:
Focus: Update teaching methods and materials based on new anatomical insights, ensuring that instruction remains relevant and effective.
Examples: Use anatomical cues, updated modifications, and evidence-based practices in your teaching approach.

Continuing education in yoga and anatomy is crucial for advancing your practice, enhancing teaching skills, and ensuring safety and effectiveness. By engaging in specialized courses, obtaining certifications, utilizing online resources, reading relevant literature, gaining practical experience, and collaborating with professionals, you can stay informed and improve both your personal practice and teaching. Embracing ongoing learning ensures that you remain at the forefront of yoga practice and instruction, offering the best possible experience for yourself and your students.